IT

STARTS

FROM THE EGG

Unraveling The Mysteries Of Fertility Diets, Miscarriage And IVF.

Written By

Kathrine M Greger

<u>DEDICATION</u>

This book is dedicated with heavy regards to those who seek to hear the cry of a baby, you're anything but alone.

TABLE OF CONTENTS

CHAPTER SEVEN:
MEDICAL BREAKTHROUGHS
(Contemporary Innovations and Discoveries in Fertility Treatment)

Fertility Vs. Science and Technology; How Far We Have Come

Fertility vs the Future; How Far Will We Go?

CHAPTER EIGHT
CRAVING OUT YOUR STORY

(Personal Paths Through Fertility)

INTRODUCTION

What if I told that you could be a mom even at age of sixty-seven? What if told you that even after being pronounced medically unable to conceive that you can and you will conceive. It's not magic it is fact. After waiting thirty-nine years in marriage if a sixty-seven year old woman was able to birth and carry her biological child in her arms tell me why you can't? When it comes to infertility there are struggles, there are fears, and the burning desire to birth a biological child. And the annoying thing about this is that people don't understand. They don't see the silent tears, or understand the stigma of not being able to conceive even after a series of trials and they certainly don't know how it feels to be in a room full of people but still feeling alone having that emptiness in your heart that only a child can fill up.

But here's the thing there is hope. Everyday as we continue to make technological and scientific advancements in the medical field the word impossible gets a bit closer with one step at the time to being "I'm possible." *It starts from the egg* isn't your average fertility book it is a perfect cocktail of scientific research, personal stories, and hope delivered shaken but not stirred. The purpose of this book is simple, to fill your heart with hope, to make you see that someone out there understands whatever it is that you might have gone through or is going through and that on your fertility journey you're most certainly not alone. This book also let's you in on the finer details of egg health and presents you with a fertility road map.

The first section of the book lets you in on the genesis of life which is the female egg, an area that is so over looked by many but plays a vital role in fertility. Fertility will be decoded, the unforeseen struggles of miscarriage will be discussed alongside an emerging area known as the (IVF) which forms the major basis of this book. Your lifestyle choices or "life habits" as I like to call them will be examined all the way to your fertility diets or nutrition taking into consideration whatever it is that will boost your chances of conception leaving no stone unturned and a personal letter from me to you is contained in this book.

The best way to maximize the benefits of this book is to treat it as you would an examination book. Set out time daily to read, keep your writing materials beside you to jot down helpful points, don't try to read it all at once but start with one chapter per-day and most importantly keep hope in your heart and have an open mind because you're not alone on this fertility journey. Despite the plethora of confusion and myths that surround conception and fertility today be rest assured that your are not alone and no matter how dire you think your situation is, it cannot be the worst possible situation out there. With this in mind allow me to welcome you to your first page on this book and invite you to come with me as we embrace creation and unravel the wonders of modern medical science together.

It Starts From The Egg

CHAPTER ONE
Genesis of Life :
(The Incredible Journey of an Egg)

In the words of the fairy godmother from one of my daughter's favorite shows as a child, Cinderella, *"even miracles take a little time"* What greater miracle is there than the miracle of life itself? Everything that is and ever will be birthed comes from the egg. And it's funny how the egg is one of the most overlooked biological components despite playing an immense role in the creation of life. The creation of life through an egg is a testament that life must go on and a process of absolute beauty to witness life from within. But I don't mean chicken eggs here, nope, I mean ones of a higher quality the ones that only biological female beings can produce, I'm talking about the egg of fertilization.

Now, if there's one thing I have noticed is that people only pay the majority of their attention to the embryo and that's only when it starts to develop, Not many people ask questions like What about the egg? Do I need to treat the egg especially before I conceive? Are there any activities that I would engage in that would prove harmful to the eggs pre and post-fertilization? Or would my general lifestyle as a whole harm the egg fertilization and development process? Not many people ask these questions and most are only focused on their trimester periods and their antenatal sessions, pregnancy nutrition, and all whatnot. Don't get me wrong these are pretty important hands down, but there's a reason why this chapter is called Life's Genesis It is because for us to understand all there is about the component of life (the egg) we must start at the very beginning. Here the biological journey of an egg will be unveiled to you and the words conception and fertilization will be elaborated in the simplest of terms, Here's a little brain teaser as we proceed. Do these two words point to the same thing or are they different entities on their own?

From Creation to Fertilization

Let's start with the basis and answer the simple question, How does the egg come about? If you remember correctly in your biology classes back in high school a particular topic that most kids with hormones flying all over the place were eager to learn about was the topic of 'reproduction.' The pre-requisite for reproduction is that you hit the puberty clock and when you hit that, eggs are going start getting produced as a woman, and then comes the painful part called menstruation(because obviously as a teen who isn't ready to settle down your eggs are pretty much non-useful to you). That's a simple summary of the egg synopsis now let's talk science a bit. You have all the eggs you will ever have when you are born. This is so because you don't produce any new eggs during your life, the most eggs you've ever had were when you were a 20-week-old female fetus, which has roughly seven million eggs. This quantity is approximately two million when you are born, and by the time you hit adolescence and start menstruating (getting periods), you will only have between 300,000 and 500,000 eggs left. You will still have 1,000 to 2,000 eggs when you reach menopause. Additionally, because these eggs are exposed to everything you are during your existence, their quality degrades as you age.

However, the fact that your egg supply is gradually diminishing need not worry you because it is a natural and ongoing process that is unaffected by birth control pills, pregnancies, nutritional supplements, or even your health or way of life. Your 20s through mid-30s are when you are most fertile. After age 35, fertility rates start to decline till menopause. Natural conception is not feasible after menopause.

One of your eggs grows and matures during the majority of menstrual cycles, enabling it to be released from an ovary (ovulation) in readiness for fertilization. However, you need many eggs to start the process before one excellent mature egg can grow. Even if hundreds of eggs are laid together, only one ovulates. The remaining eggs will disappear. Your ovaries will discharge roughly 500 mature eggs throughout a lifetime. Your ovaries will stop producing estrogen when your egg supply is exhausted, and then you will experience menopause. The majority of women experience this around the age of 50; in the industrialized world, the average age is 51.4 years. You won't be able to become pregnant naturally after this stage.

Sounds a bit scary right? I know been there, but everything that has a beginning must have an end. Now, you see why much emphasis is placed on the female egg and when you think about it, it is the only way, ever recorded through which life can come into this world. The powerful men and women of both historical and contemporary times come from an egg and even you reading this comes from one as well as the rest of us (though I'm pretty sure you're one of the cuter ones, and yes I giggled a bit here).

The above is a brief synopsis that answers the question of how the eggs came to be. And it pointed out the dawn of the creation of eggs to its dusk which is menopause. Now comes the fertilization process.

Fertilization 101

To be clear when we say fertilization here we don't mean the type that takes place in the interaction between plants and manure in the farming fields it's more complex. We mean fertilization as it relates to humans, and based on this we ask the question What is fertilization? And how does a person know that their eggs have been fertilized? Call it fertilization, call it reproduction, it still pretty much means the same thing and the end product of fertilization or reproduction there-off is the birth of new life(that is so long as there is no interruption in the whole birthing process).

So, what precisely is fertilization? The primary nucleus of an embryo is created by the joining of a sperm nucleus of paternal origin and an egg nucleus of maternal origin. In reality, the process of fertilization in all organisms involves the union of the genetic material from two gametes, or separate sex cells, each of which *consists* of half the amount of chromosomes typical for the species.

In bacteria and protozoans, the most basic type of fertilization takes place when two cells exchange genetic material.

Some people would call this process the plain word 'sex' It is sex no doubt but it is much more complex than just plain sex. I call it the intimate union that breeds life on earth and without it, the world would whither away. From the explanation given on fertilization, we are clear on the fact that through fertilization the egg which eventually becomes a child acquires the characteristics of both the father and the mother and this goes deeper than just physical traits it goes down to biological traits as well. I will give you a simple illustration of me, Mom for instance, Is off average height and hairy and my Dad on the other hand is over six feet tall but he's lacking heavily in the hair department—Then I came along I'd like to say I took the best of both worlds, long silky hair from my mom and a perfect height from my dad. And that's all there is, that is what fertilization does to the egg it gives it the biological traits from both the maternal and paternal hereditary materials.

The merging of the two gametes' membranes, which causes the creation of a channel that allows genetic material to flow from one cell to the other, is the first critical event in fertilization. For instance, pollination, which occurs before fertilization in advanced plants, is when pollen is carried to and comes into contact with the female gamete or macrospore. In advanced species, fusion is typically followed by a single spermatozoon penetrating the egg. A cell (zygote) created after conception is capable of cell division to create an entirely new person

It looks pretty interesting to unravel the general dynamics behind fertilization but we are talking about humans in this context. And yes, the answer to my little brain teaser earlier is that both fertilization and conception mean the same thing. As was previously said, sperm and an egg combine during conception (or fertilization). It's but one of a plethora of events that lead to conception. Menstruation and conception are closely connected processes.

A menstrual cycle is a term used to describe the sequence of events that occur in your body each month as it prepares for the possibility of conception. Both women and people who were assigned the gender of a female at birth (AFAB) experience ovulation during the menstrual cycle. Your ovary releases an egg for fertilization during ovulation. Fimbriae, which are teeny, finger-like organs, aid in directing the egg through your fallopian tubes and into your uterus. An egg may become fertilized by a sperm during this passage through your fallopian tubes. In the testicles of men or those who were assigned male at birth (AMAB), sperm production begins. Millions of sperm cells are released during ejaculation with the sole intent of locating an egg to fertilize. Sperm cells swim up through your vagina and into your fallopian tubes during unprotected sex. Only one sperm manages to fertilize an egg despite millions of sperm competing to reach and enter the egg. Eggs disintegrate if sperm cannot fertilize them.

A fertilized egg, also known as a zygote, continues to travel down your fallopian tube if a sperm is successful in its attempt to fertilize an egg. As it does so, it divides into two cells, then four cells, then more cells as it travels. The zygote arrives in your uterus about a week after the sperm and egg are fertilized—It then morphs into a blastocyst, a conglomerate of roughly a hundred developing cells. The blastocyst then adheres to the endometrium, the lining of your uterus. This process of attachment is known as "implantation." However, only because conception takes place does not guarantee implantation. Occasionally, implantation fails, and the fertilized egg is passed during your subsequent menstrual cycle.

If implantation occurs, the cells keep dividing; some become your baby while others become the placenta. You start to exude hormones that alert your body that a child is developing inside your womb. These hormones have to instruct the uterus to maintain its lining in place against shedding it. This means that you won't get a period, which may be how you find out you are pregnant for the first time. If you're wondering how to be certain you're fertilized, it's simple—just get tested.

The fertilized egg passes via your fallopian tubes to reach your uterus following fertilization. The fertilized egg, also known as an embryo, attaches to the uterine wall. The placenta begins to develop as a result. Human chorionic gonadotropin (HCG for short) starts to be made by your placenta and released into your blood and urine. At this moment, which is visible about 11 days after conception, it's time to break out the pregnancy toolkit and take the test that will tell if you'll be referred to as a mommy in nine months. Our next line of action here is to look at the biological journey of an egg in a bid to find out what becomes of said egg after the fertilization has taken place

The Biological Journey of an Egg

We have looked at the egg from the angle of creation to fertilization now we ask the question, what does the biological journey of an egg look like? In the event of successful fertilization, the next process that occurs here is the life process. Remember, that we mentioned earlier that the end product of fertilization of the eggs is called 'life' nothing too fancy or complex just life.

The biological journey of an egg can be captured in three simple stages called the 'three stages of fetal development.' Fetal development is a meticulous and well-organized procedure. It starts before you even realize you're pregnant and concludes when your baby is born.

Between conception and delivery, several intricate steps must be taken. There are three stages of fetal development: germinal, embryonic, and fetal. Although most individuals don't discuss these terms during pregnancy, being aware of them can be useful.

Germinal stage

The sperm and egg unite in your fallopian tube to form a zygote, which begins its one-week journey down to your uterus. During this journey, the zygote divides numerous times to eventually create two separate structures: one structure becomes the embryo (and later, the fetus), and the other becomes the placenta. This is the germinal stage, which is the shortest stage of fetal development. At this stage, a successful implantation only means one thing no more periods for you at least for the next nine months.

Embryonic stage

From roughly the third week of pregnancy to the eighth week of pregnancy, exists the time frame for the embryonic stage. Beginning to resemble a human is the blastocyst—It is currently referred to as an embryo. The neural tube, which later gives rise to the head, eyes, mouth, and limbs, as well as the brain and spinal cord, starts to take shape. Around the sixth week, the embryo's heart begins to grow and pulse. Around the sixth week, buds that will grow into limbs and legs also start to form. The majority of the embryo's organs and systems are formed by the end of the eighth week. This is the time in most women's pregnancies when morning sickness starts.

Fetal stage

The fetal stage of development begins in the ninth week of pregnancy and lasts until delivery. The embryo now formally develops into a fetus at this point. The fetus begins to show signs of its assigned sex at nine weeks into the pregnancy, though your healthcare provider cannot yet see it on ultrasound. Major body systems and organs continue to develop and grow in the fetus—the things that grow at this point include fingernails, hair, and eyelashes. The fetus can move, even though you might not feel it until 20 weeks into your pregnancy. In the fetal stage, the majority of growth—both in weight and length—occurs.

And dear readers there you have it the journey of an egg. In this brief chapter, we have successfully talked about what the egg is, and how it relates to females. How it relates to the concepts of creation and fertilization and the biological journey that it takes until it produces life. Have you ever heard of the term 'decoding fertility' before? I guess not let you but more in-depth unraveling more mysteries in the next chapter, it's more exciting than the preliminaries and I promise to be with you every step of the way.

CHAPTER TWO
The Art of Decoding Fertility:
(All you need to know about Egg Quality and its Influence)

In the words of Robert Ludlum *"Hope is the only thing stronger than fear."* While most people never consider the quality of their eggs before pregnancy, those who do are more often than not faced with a harsh question laced with fear and the question is, are my eggs good enough for fertilization? I tell you this fear not and let the pages of this chapter fill you with hope.

In the previous chapter, we talked about what an egg is and its relationship to fertilization was our paramount point of focus. We referred to the dawn and dusk of eggs, the estimated number of eggs that a female has and produces throughout their life until they hits menopause, and the journey that an egg goes through before it produces life. In this chapter, we are going to go a bit more in-depth and discuss a very neglected part of pregnancy and that's about the quality of the egg that is yet to be fertilized.

There is no doubt that medical technology has made significant improvements over the past decade in the art of aiding fertility, but we ask a simple question What good is the addition of a component when the source itself is of no use? I will give you a little illustration, I once came across someone who was in dire need of an intravenous injection since oral drips and pills were no good to alleviate his situation, The best option here was to go for the intravenous but when the injection was administered not only was there a failure to find a vein it was also discovered that he had collapsed veins due to substance intake making intravenous nigh impossible.

The reason for giving this illustration is this, What use would it be to try and get fertilized or conceive when the quality of your eggs is as low as low can be, Wouldn't it be the same as wasting water on the proverbial duck's back? This chapter takes you deeper into the world of egg quality before and after fertilization. Here we ask the questions, What is egg quality and why is it so important? What happens if your egg quality is low? What affects your egg quality? What showcases poor egg quality? And how can one improve said egg quality?

The Role of Egg Quality in Pregnancy and Conception

The egg quality is the overall biological health of an egg before and after fertilization. This takes into account various factors like the health of the egg, and the biological capacity of the egg to withstand fertilization and see it through to the end. Did you know that the quality of an egg is so important that it plays a role even in serious cases like miscarriages, fetal development, and other health issues like genetic deformities and whatnot?

When we say that we are decoding fertility here we are simply breaking down the structural integrity of an egg's quality to ascertain ways to improve it and avoid ways that would lead to a downgrade in egg quality. The quality of the egg, or oocyte as it is sometimes written, is crucial to the success of reproductive treatments. What does this signify, though? It means, therefore, that having eggs of greater quality increases the likelihood that they will be fertilized, grow into an embryo, implant in the uterus, and then result in pregnancy. The primary oocyte (egg), which involves cell division and maturity before ovulation, occasionally experiences due-process mistakes(anomalies) that result in genetic defects in the egg. Poorer egg quality is one of these anomalies. Thus, you will find that it may be more challenging for women whose eggs are of lower quality to become pregnant.

One essential requirement for fertilization and pregnancy to result in a healthy birth is the quality of the eggs needed to conceive spontaneously or with the fertility-assisted (IVF) procedure. This mostly has to do with the expecting mother's egg supply. One of the elements that reduces the likelihood of conception is the mother's ovarian reserve (AMH) not having enough eggs.

Women have a specific amount of egg reserve when they are born. In other words, the reproductive cell egg is not produced by the female body. When a person reaches puberty, which is regarded as the start of the fertile period, they typically have 400 thousand eggs—Every month, one egg is released into the fallopian tubes during the menstrual cycle, although the person loses roughly 1000 eggs each month. But as people become older, this loss gets worse. When a person is 40 years old, only 3% of the eggs that were in their ovarian reserve when they were 30 years old are still there. The quality of the eggs declines as the quantity of eggs in the ovarian reserve declines. In other words, the likelihood of conceiving naturally is significantly decreased beyond the age of 40.

To put this in plain simple words the lower the quality of your eggs is the lower the chances of you getting called Mommy by your biological child(if you're a first-time mother). If the quality of your eggs is low then the higher the chances of a miscarriage or a birth defect. And to make matters even worse if you are engaging in activities or ingesting different foods that don't bid well for your egg quality and overall body(like being a junk food freak) then we might have to announce and crown said person as the new duchess of barren's Ville, but that's not going to happen as fertility is the goal in this chapter and we are going to be looking at next is what affects the potential quality of eggs before and after fertilization occurs.

Factors Impacting the Overall Egg Quality of a Female

As with everything in the world, there is always the positive and the negative side of things. Of what use would it be for us to talk about egg quality without talking about its positive and negative aspects? Let's take age for instance, most people dream of getting older and living longer but are you also aware that age is one of the determining factors of egg quality? Didn't see that coming huh? Before we jump the gun on this and start spitting words about good and bad egg quality here's my advice to you, go run a test. The essence of the test here is to determine the current state of your egg quality and help point you to the next course of action to take, If your eggs are of top quality then that's a sign that you're on the right track, if they are not you have to cut down certain habits and do whatever it takes to improve your egg quality before you start trying to conceive in the first place. Below is a list of some of the egg quality tests that you could run to determine the state of your eggs;

- Day 3 FSH and Estradiol

- Trans-vaginal Ultrasound

- Clomid Challenge

- Anti-Mullerian Hormone (AMH)

The tests aren't limited to these but these are the most potent ones that there is. Once done with these tests we can now start the business of listing out those factors or signs of negative egg quality.

An unnaturally high chromosomal count

One indication of poor egg quality may be an abnormally high number of chromosomes. An egg typically contains 23 chromosomes. The resulting embryo will have 46 chromosomes, which is the typical number, after being fertilized by a sperm (which also contains 23 chromosomes). When the chromosomes are normal, the egg quality is also normal. The number of chromosomes will be less or higher than normal if the eggs are defective or of poor quality. Aneuploid eggs are what these are known as. If this egg is used for fertilization, the embryo that develops will have an unusually high number of chromosomes.

Chromosome disorder problems

Chromosomes are DNA structures linked to proteins; they also house an organism's genome, which is its genetic makeup. One indication of poor egg quality could be a chromosomal abnormality. Aneuploid eggs are frequently produced in greater quantities as a woman gets older. Chromosome problems, such as those with extra copies of chromosomes or defective chromosomes, may develop from this anomaly and it can therefore be an indication of low egg quality.

Low FSH reserves

Follicle Stimulating Hormone (FSH) is a hormone secreted by the pituitary gland that tells the ovaries to release an egg every cycle. As the egg quality declines, the ovaries become more resistant to FSH, which makes it necessary for the body to produce more FSH. This results in higher levels of FSH in the body (and low FSH reserves), which is one of the signs of poor egg quality and will be taken into account.

Low levels of estradiol

When E2 levels rise the ovarian follicles are stimulated to grow; if the E2 levels are high at an early stage of the cycle, it can indicate that the eggs are of lower quality and that the ovaries are releasing them earlier than expected. Low levels of estradiol are also one of the signs of poor egg quality since estradiol is the hormone that happens to communicate signals from the ovaries to the brain.

Low levels of anti-mullerian hormone (AMH)

AMH levels that are low could be one indication of poor egg quality. The cells of eggs secrete AMH, a glycoprotein, during the early stages of egg formation. It promotes the maturation of the eggs and aids in their development. One of the earliest indicators is the AMH level, which falls before the FSH levels rise. Low AMH, which is directly produced by the ovaries as opposed to FSH, which is produced in the pituitary gland, is one of the primary indicators of poor egg quality. When deciding how to improve egg quality, low levels of AMH may point to problems with the eggs' quality in an egg quality test.

Low follicle count

One indication of poor egg quality may be a low follicle count. This can be discovered via transvaginal ultrasound, which counts the number of follicles in the ovaries that are between four and nine millimeters in diameter. Fewer follicles could mean that there are issues with the amount and quality of eggs.

Irregular menstrual cycles and trouble getting pregnant

It can be an indicator of poor egg quality if you are having trouble conceiving and haven't been successful for some time. Menstrual period irregularities or extremely extended cycles may be signs of ovulation problems. These can happen when the eggs do not reach the ovulation phase because they are not developing properly or because they are of lower quality.

Miscarriages

Multiple miscarriages may be a sign of poor egg quality, which is one of the more unpleasant aspects. It can mean that the eggs being generated are abnormal or aneuploid. Although such fetuses are typically prevented from implanting in the uterus, defective eggs nonetheless have a chance of doing so—Such circumstances could lead to a miscarriage. A miscarriage can be caused by a variety of things. Given this information, it should come as no surprise that a history of multiple miscarriages may be a warning sign of poor egg quality.

Irregular use of antibodies

When antibiotics are used erratically and without a doctor's prescription, it disturbs the vaginal flora in women and makes fungal infections more likely to develop. This lessens the capacity of sperm, the male reproductive cell, to be confined and thus lessens the likelihood that the egg will be fertilized or that the fertilized egg will be able to adhere to the uterus. Despite this, it's crucial to note that antibiotic medications used for doctor control don't harm the quality of eggs. I hope this acts as a wake-up call for some women because females who are fond of using antibiotics irregularly are mostly to blame for this aspect.

Stress

Yes, stress Let's talk about stress, think of it like this if extreme stress is enough to cause drastic factors like death it would be a pipe dream to assume that it can't affect egg quality. Stress by itself may be a sufficient cause of infertility. Avoiding stress is crucial because of this. Alcohol, nicotine, and caffeine usage all have a deleterious impacts on ovarian quality while not affecting stress levels. Put another way, if the other variables were wrestlers, stress would be the world heavyweight champion, dominating even important variables like the age of the involved female as stress can make us appear older than we are.

Gosh! That was a very long list and that's not even all of it, but as always I bring to you the most important factors and signs of them all. Now it is time we turned our gazes to the light at the end of the tunnel as we answer the question How do we improve egg quality?

How to Improve Your Egg Quality

Taking age and other biological defects from family out the window that may or may not affect the quality of your eggs, your best bet is following the methods mentioned below as ways to improve your egg quality and boost fertilization. The reason why we took out age and family-based biological factors is that those are they two factors that no one can do anything about or find ways to improve on they are just there and affixed like that. It's like advising a woman who is eighty years old on how to get pregnant at eight-five which is impossible by all standards. Thus without further ado, I present to you the ways to improve your egg quality and they include;

Being healthy in terms of weight

Your body mass index (BMI) should be as healthy as possible. Your fertility and the quality of your eggs are both affected by excess weight. Also, your hormonal balance is impacted by obesity, which might prevent ovulation. By reducing inflammation (which otherwise lowers blood flow to the ovaries) and harmonizing your reproductive hormones, a high-fat, low-carb diet boosts overall fertility and egg quality. Fat also aids in conception by providing your body with the energy and support for fetal cell growth.

Dealing with stress effectively

Your body releases stress-related hormones like cortisol and prolactin, which prevent you from laying eggs. A session of yoga or meditation practice, light exercise like strolling, and relaxing warm baths are all excellent strategies to reduce unhealthy stress levels. These also balance your immune system and promote blood flow to your reproductive organs.

Eat nutritious meals

Eating nutrient-dense foods improves the health and quality of eggs. To provide your body the nutrients it needs to nourish your eggs, include healthy grains, lean meats, leafy greens, fresh vegetables, fruit, and nuts in your diet. When possible, stay away from processed foods and meats, and keep your salt and sugar intake in check.

Adding to your diet

Think about taking fish oil (Omega 3s), melatonin, and coenzyme Q10. The antioxidants in these supplements enhance ovarian health, improve sleep quality, and improve egg quality. While Q10 supplies antioxidants that help your mitochondria, omega 3s maintain fertility and improve egg quality. This gives your body the energy it needs to carry out DNA replication to improve the generation of high-quality eggs. Vitamin E increases follicular blood flow, which is important for producing high-quality eggs, and vitamin A reduces oxidative stress. Vitamin A also improves oocyte quality and embryo development.

Get a good night's sleep

Even while it might not seem like much, rest has a direct impact on egg quality and fertility. Your body can repair cells, regain energy, and release hormones like melatonin thanks to it. Melatonin is essential for reproductive processes because it promotes healthy oocyte development, ovulation, and embryo development. This allows your body to produce high-quality, healthy eggs. This is especially beneficial because melatonin production in women after the age of 40 declines.

Improve your blood flow

Better egg health is achieved by generating oxygen-rich blood flow to the organism. It's a good idea to drink a lot of water (preferably 64 ounces per day) to prevent dehydration. Yoga positions including the reclining hero, child, and lotus can also increase blood flow

Avoid cigarettes:

Unless you're planning to join the X-men soon I suggest you take cigarettes off the table. Cigarettes contain chemicals that can alter the DNA of your egg cells, rendering them useless for fertilization and accelerating the loss of eggs from your ovaries.

Freeze your eggs now

If any of these ways seem a bit over the top to you then your best bet and last resort is to go all Dr. Freeze on your eggs. Since your egg quality declines with age, freezing your eggs is done to ensure their greatest quality and conception possibilities. By cryopreserving your eggs now, you can prevent that from happening and ensure that they maintain the same degree of health and quality as the day they were frozen.

At the end of this chapter, I think it fair to state the basis first doing an egg quality test would help steer you in the right direction on your pregnancy quest, then Based on the result offered to you by your doctor you can then avoid any and all things or activities that would reduce the quality of your eggs and stick to those that would improve said quality. If even these simple steps prove a bit over the top for you then your best and last resort is to freeze your eggs in their highest form and use them when ready to conceive(but I warn you though this doesn't come cheap).

CHAPTER THREE
The Unforeseen Struggle
(Understanding the Concept of Miscarriage)

I spent a greater part of my day pacing around the house before writing this chapter since it is a topic that hits a little too close to home. To be honest I didn't know how to begin, what to say, how to turn inwards and pour out the emotions buried deep and lay it out on a canvas of white as we talk about the concept of miscarriages, but I did promise that I'd be here till the end with you reading this right now so…let's begin.

In this chapter, our major sense of focus is on the concept of miscarriages. How they happen? What it is? What signs it brings? What does it leave behind in the wake of its aftermath? And the relationship that it shares with the quality of the eggs before and after fertilization. Miscarriage is and will always be one of the nightmares of an expecting mother. It is heavily tethered to the feeling of what could have been. Sure, people die everyday it is as normal as normal can be when we reach the end of our biological composition we expire and die but what makes miscarriage especially painful is the fact that the being that dies doesn't even get the chance to live in the first place.

What could have been, how they could have looked when they grew up, what type of talent could they have had if they were born and who would they take after more, Mom or Dad? These are the thoughts that hover around my mind at the mention of the word miscarriage. It is an irreplaceable loss to a mother so much so that even if she has another perfectly healthy child she still can't help but wonder what could have been had the child lived.

These are the silent battles of an expecting mother after they have gone through the cold hands of miscarriage before. We find that miscarriage is a bit of a taboo topic and not many people like to talk about it more so than the expecting mother herself— it's almost like the way people view serious illnesses like cancer or aids no one wants to talk about them they just want to be treated and move one. Health reports have shown that psychologically by experiencing miscarriage some expecting mothers felt like they were a part of some secret society that no one talk them that miscarriage was their membership pass. Some even felt like they were spiritually punished for their wrong deeds and a whole lot of other emotional cracks.

In addition to talking about the earlier mentioned areas we will point out some common misconception about miscarriage and answer the question does miscarriage leave behind emotional scars in its wake on the couple or couples who experience it?

Let's begin, shall we?

Miscarriage 101

No matter what definition you see or hear within and beyond the pages of this book and other books on miscarriage it simply means a loss, a loss of life, and a future potential (what could have been). A miscarriage (also known as a spontaneous abortion) is the unintended termination of a pregnancy within the first 20 weeks of gestation. A "miscarriage" does not necessarily mean that carrying the pregnancy to term was sinful.

The majority of miscarriages are unavoidable and happen when the fetus stops developing. Let there never be a time that you feel as an expecting mother that you're the cause of your miscarriage it happens as a result of factors beyond your control, not your fault although it is important to note that certain factors like your age, egg quality and the lifestyle you live can cause or facilitate your chances of experiencing miscarriage. Even after keeping these factors in mind. You still have to be watchful of certain signs that might herald a miscarriage.

Although 15% of pregnancies, according to health professionals, result in a miscarriage, you shouldn't let this worry you because your risk of pregnancy loss decreases each week you are pregnant. Miscarriages occur in about 15% of pregnancies. The risk of miscarriage in the second trimester (13–19 weeks) ranges from 1% to 5%. The chance of miscarriage is influenced by a number of variables, including your age and health. However, if the expectant mother does not have any additional medical issues, everyone's risk of miscarriage decreases each week of pregnancy.

Let's dive a bit deeper at this point, and ponder on certain factors like what are the signs of a miscarriage? What causes miscarriages? And what types of miscarriages are there?

Causes of a Miscarriage

According to medical professionals, the majority of miscarriages are brought on by incorrect chromosomes, which are the fundamental units governing a baby's growth. Babies who have an imbalance of chromosomes will not develop normally. About 50% of miscarriages in the first trimester (up to 13 weeks of pregnancy) are brought on by chromosomal abnormalities (Chromosomes, which are tiny constructs located inside the cells of your body, carry your genes).

All of a person's physical characteristics, including sex preference, blood type, and hair and eye color, are determined by genes. Two sets of chromosomes combine when the egg and sperm unite during fertilization. A fetus will have an abnormal number of chromosomes if an egg or sperm contains more or less than usual. A fertilized egg's cells divide and multiply multiple times as it develops into a fetus. This process can go wrong and result in miscarriage. The majority of chromosomal issues are accidental. The exact cause of this is unknown.

Other factors that cause miscarriage include;
- Negative life habits like such as excessive smoking, drinking alcohol or over abusing recreational drugs.
- Disorders of the immune system like lupus.
- Severe kidney disease.
- Hormonal imbalances.
- Age.
- Infection.

Having pointed these our when then ask the question what are the signs of a miscarriage?

Signs of a Miscarriage

By signs in this context we don't mean looking out for signs that appear when the miscarriage is already taking place but also looking out for signs that occurs before miscarriage even takes place and at the first instance of these signs the best line of action is to immediately contact your health provider.

The reason for this is that you might not even know when the miscarriage occurs sometimes so it's best to be safe than sorry. Some of these signs include;

- progressive bleeding from light to heavy. Blood clots or grey tissue may also flow through you.
- stomach discomfort and cramps (which are typically stronger than menstruation cramps).
- Severe mid or lower back pain is possible.
- A decrease in pregnancy symptoms.

Types of Miscarriage

The types of miscarriages play a vital role in aid your health provider determine the type of treatment that would be given in the event of a miscarriage and they include;

Missed miscarriage: In this case, you lost the pregnancy but are ignorant of it. An ultrasound reveals that the fetus has no heartbeat even if there are no symptoms of miscarriage.

Complete miscarriage: In this kind of miscarriage, the pregnancy has been lost, and your uterus is now empty. Both bleeding and fetal tissue have already passed through you at this stage. Your healthcare provider might use an ultrasound to confirm if it is a complete miscarriage.

Recurrent miscarriage: This entails three miscarriages that occur back-to-back in quick succession. The sole benefit of this, however, is that it only occurs in around 1% of marriages because it is so uncommon.

Threatened miscarriage: Here you'd find that your cervix remains closed during a possible miscarriage, yet you bleed and have cramps in your pelvis. Typically, the pregnancy ends without any more issues. Your doctor may monitor you more closely the rest of your pregnancy.

Inevitable miscarriage: This is the more terrifying type of miscarriage; you will bleed, cramp, and your cervix will have begun to dilate. Amniotic fluid may leak from you. It's possible to miscarry completely.

Common Mythical Misconceptions about Miscarriage

Would you believe it if I told you that some people attribute a miscarriage to a witch attack or to Karma. Bet you never saw that coming eh? These are some of the common misconception of miscarriages and they are no jokes. Health and psychological experts state that in the state of extreme loss caused by miscarriage couples go into heavy grief and are eager to believe anything to give them some sort of closure and help alleviate their pain.

These beliefs give birth to these myths that surround miscarriages. Some mothers blame themselves thinking thoughts like oh, if only I had eaten more healthy meals, if only I had slept more, had relaxed more or done this and done that more— it generally gives birth to that feeling of inward guilt on the part of the mother. Below are a few of the common misconceptions and popular myths of miscarriage;

Miscarriages can't ever be prevented.

Well answering this would be a yes and a no. The thing is, miscarriages are factors that are beyond the control of anyone, but there are certain things that can be done to lessen and also things that can be done to increase the risk of a miscarriage. Let's take smoking for instance, an expecting mother that smokes 10 packs of cigarettes a day even during her trimesters has a higher risk of a miscarriage than an expecting mother who doesn't smoke at all or quits smoking at the instance of her pregnancy.

You have to wait 3 months after a miscarriage to try and conceive again.

According to a recent health study, you can conceive as soon as one month after a miscarriage and still have a healthy, full-term pregnancy. Women are always advised by health professionals to wait until their blood test value (serum beta-hCG) drops to zero before attempting again; this could happen as soon as a few weeks or even a month. However, some medical professionals might suggest waiting longer if a woman had a procedure known as a suction D&C (dilation and curettage) after the miscarriage.

Spotting or bleeding during pregnancy means you're having a miscarriage.

If you're a first time mother then it is my humble advice that you don't panic when you see yourself bleeding during your first trimester. Don't be scared but understand that first, bleeding is very common during the pregnancies 20% to 40% of women bleed during pregnancies and even very healthy pregnancies experience bleeding from time to time. Secondly, in the event of bleeding don't get scared instead report to your health provider immediately and have them run a few tests to ascertain your condition.

Having one miscarriage means you're likely to have another.

This particular myths is born from sheer paranoia. Having one miscarriage does not put you at risk of having another. One miscarriage should not completely choke out your optimistic spirit and discourage you from trying again although this is easier said than done but it is plausible. However, Health experts report that having two miscarriages in frequent successions is a clear sign that you need to get yourself medically checked to ascertain the problem.

Miscarriages are caused by supernatural forces

(OK I'ii admit it this is the only part of this chapter that got me laughing hard) it is true that most of us are very spiritual and thus belief in the supernatural it's fine I respect that but unless you have like some ancient family curse like the curse of La Llorona on you or you vividly offended the creator by some action of yours(at this point you just know you're screwed) then I kindly suggest that no matter the amount of pain and thinking that miscarriage cause never think that you're cursed or that something supernatural is after you it doesn't help and people might think you delusional. Do the best you can as an expecting mother and watch everything thing go well for you without fail.

Emotional Effects of Miscarriage on Couples

In my younger years in 2007 I used to have this Aunt of mine who was very love-able and had a cheerful personality let's call her Aunt E. Aunt E used to be one of my favorites well, at least she was until that fateful event. She had a miscarriage and when that happened she and her husband took it really hard. They first had slight issues between themselves when the grief of the loss hit them but the worst part came after they sorted out their issues they withdrew from everyone, and I mean everyone including my family.

My aunt first started by returning my mom's old clothes and other stuff that she had given to her freely in the early 2000s, she did the same to everyone else and finally she and her husband moved away to another vicinity entirely. It hurt alot but then I couldn't understand the state of their grief — eventually some years later they had more kids (two to be exact) but things were never the same again between us I'd like to think that it was their personal decision that caused this but I'd be kidding myself if I didn't know that the root cause of it all was the loss of their first child. People don't always know the depth of the problems of others or even take said problem seriously until it hits close to home then they start to understand the pain of others. After pointing that out below are some of the effects of miscarriage on couples;

Emotional effects: There are major emotional problems for both parents. Clearly, both prospective parents are experiencing a genuine sense of loss. It can be devastating to have your hopes of becoming a parent dashed, as it was for Aunt E. Both of you could be nervous about getting pregnant again because you don't want to take a chance on experiencing the physical and psychological toll of a miscarriage. A mother's sense of emptiness is both emotional and physical. Feelings of failure or guilt could exist. Additionally, there might be a general feeling of despair or discouragement.

Relationship effects: At this time, you and your partner both need emotional support, which may strain your marriage. It is simple to get guilty and place blame. Tensions and minor irritations can worsen. You might even think that your relationship is about to end.

Physical effects: A miscarriage has a lot of unpleasant and painful consequences for the mother. Large clots and considerable vaginal bleeding are typically present. The mother and her partner find this a little unsettling on its own. How much blood or how many clots, after all, is too much? How can you distinguish between what is normal and what is not? A mother's body also frequently responds the same way it does before she gives birth, thus, for instance, her breasts may expand and become painful. Her hormones will probably result in unforeseen emotional and physical responses, which will only make the feelings of loss more difficult.

There's even a spiritual effect where people who were believers tend to stray away after the miscarriage and lose their faith but that's by the way. As we proceed to the next chapter we dedicate this chapter to everyone who has ever had a painful miscarriage and encourage that they should never be devoid of hope.

CHAPTER FOUR
A Scientific Miracle
(Deep Dive into in-vitro Fertilization)

Now, what is a miracle? it is an event or an act that goes beyond the rational understanding of humans. To be clear it's not magic those are tricks for entertainment but it is something spectacular to witness. Imagine being told that you might be not be able to conceive and this causes you to lose all hope but yet through the innovations of science and technology a way is opened for you and your hope is reignited once more that is what in-vitro fertilization (IVF) does for a couple who has lost all hope of conception.

You have probably been hearing stories about women who are way past their prime conceiving and giving birth, or those who give birth to perfectly healthy children despite having a long line of genetic diseases on their family tree this is one out of the many miracles of the (IVF). in this chapter we are going forge ahead and answer questions like what is the (IVF) all about? Who can do the (IVF)? why do people do it? What is the general statistics regarding it? Are there any risks associated to it? And what are some of the common myths that surround the (IVF) that we have to debunk?

One of my favorite quotes that I came across as regards to the (IVF) is that *"the miracle of life is a gift beyond measure and for those who struggle with infertility the (IVF) can make that dream a reality."* its been a while since I heard lines so beautiful and so filled with hope. Everyone deserves hope including you reading this right now and if you have an issue with conception and you're still pondering about what to do to alleviate this issue of yours why don't you sit back, put your feet up and let this chapter be your guide to clarifying any and all doubts you might have about the (IVF) process.

Without further delays let's begin now.

In-vitro Fertilization Unveiled

The difficult process of in vitro fertilization, generally known as (IVF), can result in pregnancy. It is a remedy for infertility, a disorder that prevents most couples from becoming pregnant for at least a year after attempting. (IVF) can also be used to stop a child from inheriting genetic issues. Mature eggs are removed from ovaries and fertilized by sperm in a laboratory during in vitro fertilization. One or more of the fertilized eggs are then surgically implanted in a uterus, which is where infants are developed. (IVF) cycles are completed in two to three weeks on average. When these processes are divided into separate steps, the process can sometimes take longer.

It is trite that the most successful fertility procedure that works with eggs, embryos, and sperm is in vitro fertilization. This collection of procedures is often referred to as assisted reproductive technology. The eggs and sperm from the pair can be used for (IVF). It could also involve sperm, eggs, or embryos from a known or unidentified donor. Sometimes a woman who has had an embryo implanted in her uterus is used as a fetal carrier.

Always keep in mind though that your odds of conceiving a healthy child with (IVF) will be influenced by a number of factors, including your age and the cause of your infertility, in addition to many more. Additionally, (IVF) requires receiving treatments that can be pricey, intrusive, and time-consuming. The (IVF) Is a procedure so complex that it makes multiple pregnancies possible if more than one embryo is implanted in the uterus.

You ever heard the term *"test tube babes"* before? They get this term from the (IVF) process. In vitro fertilization (IVF) is a form of assisted reproduction that is used to treat infertility, facilitate gestational surrogacy, and, when combined with pre-implantation genetic screening, prevent the transmission of genetic disorders. (IVF) babies are most commonly referred to as test tube babies.

Some people even go as far as calling it the artificial baby creation system but that's by the way, people can call the (IVF) what they please but it doesn't change the fact that its innovation in the area of fertility is nothing short of impeccable. So now we know a bit more of what the the (IVF) is all about the next big question to answer is why the (IVF)?

Why the (IVF)?

Well not to state the obvious but it is called in-vitro fertilization for a reason so the big ole answer to this is "fertility." For a couple who finds it hard to conceive after series of trials the (IVF) is your best bet yet(just make sure your pocket can carry its weight though). You and your spouse might be able to attempt various treatment options that require fewer or no procedures that enter the body before doing (IVF) to address infertility. For instance, fertility medications can stimulate egg production in the ovaries.

And a process known as intrauterine insemination, often known as ovulation, involves injecting sperm straight into the uterus. The (IVF) procedure may not only be used to treat severe infertility but also to increase a couple's fertility and to help them if either of them suffers from the conditions stated below;

Fallopian tube damage or blockage: The fallopian tubes carry eggs from the ovaries to the uterus. It becomes difficult for an egg to be fertilized or for an embryo to migrate to the uterus if both tubes become damaged or clogged.

Endometriosis: When uterine tissue protrudes outside of the uterus, the result is this disorder. The uterus, fallopian tubes, and ovaries are frequently impacted by endometriosis.

Previous surgery to prevent pregnancy: The fallopian tubes can be cut or blocked during a procedure known as tubal ligation to permanently end pregnancy. (IVF) may be useful if you want to get pregnant following a tubal ligation. If you don't want or are unable to have surgery to reverse tubal ligation, this can be an alternative for you.

Issues with sperm: It may be challenging for sperm to fertilize an egg if there aren't enough of them or if they undergo remarkable changes in motility, size, or shape. A visit to an infertility expert may be necessary to see whether there are any treatable abnormalities or other health concerns if sperm testing reveals problems.

Unexplained infertility: When tests are unable to determine the cause of someone's infertility, this occurs.

A genetic disorder: Your medical staff may advise obtaining an IVF procedure if you or your partner are at risk of spreading a genetic issue to your unborn child. Pre-implantation genetic testing is what it is known as. Following egg collection and fertilization, the fertilized eggs are examined for certain genetic flaws. However, not all of these illnesses are known to exist. It is possible to implant embryos into the uterus that don't appear to have any genetic issues.

A desire to preserve fertility due to cancer or other health conditions: Radiation and chemotherapy for cancer can have a negative impact on fertility. (IVF) may be a viable option for future pregnancy if you are going to begin cancer treatment. Their ovaries can be harvested for eggs, which can then be frozen for later use. Or, the eggs can be fertilized, then the embryos can be preserved for later use.

Those who lack a uterus and so require someone else to go through the (IVF) pregnancy process on their behalf..

The reasons for the (IVF) are endless but one thing is for sure the (IVF) process stands up to the challenge every time. What about the process of the (IVF) which steps and procedures are involved before the (IVF) is deemed successful.

Unraveling the (IVF) Process

For every journey or every goal that is desired there has to be a process or a procedure that must be followed to achieve said goal and the (IVF) is no different it is a miracle not magic and below is an in-depth analysis of the in-vitro fertilization process.

Birth control pills or estrogen

Your health provider could recommend estrogen or birth control pills before you begin (IVF) treatment. This controls the start of your menstrual cycle and stops the development of ovarian cysts. It enables your doctor to manage your care and increase the quantity of mature eggs collected during the egg retrieval operation. While some people are prescribed birth control pills that include both estrogen and progesterone, others only receive estrogen.

Ovarian stimulation

It is trite that during a healthy person's natural cycle who is of reproductive age, an egg batch begins to grow each month. Usually, only one egg develops to the point where it can ovulate. Then the eggs in that group that were still developing naturally disintegrate. Throughout your (IVF) cycle, you will be given injectable hormone medications to assist the batch of eggs to mature all at once and completely. This indicates that you might have numerous eggs instead of just one (as in a natural cycle). The kind, amount, and timing of your medication will be based on your medical history, age, AMH (anti-mullerian hormone) level, and response to ovarian stimulation from prior IVF cycles.

Other steps under this process include:

● Monitoring:

● Trigger shot

Egg retrieval

At this point, your doctor uses an ultrasound to direct a tiny needle into your vagina to each of your ovaries. Your eggs are extracted from each follicle using a suction equipment that is attached to the needle. Your eggs are put in a dish with a unique solution. From there the dish will be placed in a relatively safe incubator. For this surgery, light anesthesia and medication are utilized to lessen discomfort. The "trigger shot," your last hormone injection, is given 36 hours before to egg retrieval.

Fertilization

The afternoon following your egg harvesting procedure, the embryologist will attempt to fertilize all mature eggs using intracytoplasmic sperm injection, or ICSI. This implies that each developed egg will get sperm injection. ICSI cannot be conducted on immature eggs. The undeveloped eggs will be put in a dish with sperm and food. Rarely do immature eggs complete their development in the dish.

If an immature egg ultimately matures, the sperm in the dish can try to fertilize the egg. However, it is crucial to remember that 70% of mature eggs typically fertilize. For instance, seven out of ten ripe eggs will fertilize if ten are recovered. The fertilized egg will develop into an embryo if it is successful. If there are too many eggs or you don't want all of the eggs fertilized, you can freeze some of the eggs before fertilization for later use.

Embryo development

We will carefully monitor the growth of your embryos over the next five to six days. Before it can be transferred to your uterus, your embryo must clear a number of difficult obstacles. 50% of fertilized embryos make it to the blastocyst stage on average. The best time to transfer to your uterus is at this stage. Three or four of seven fertilized eggs, for instance, might progress to the blastocyst stage. Usually, 50% of the remaining candidates do not advance and are eliminated. All viable embryos will be stored in anticipation of impending embryo transfers on day five or day six following fertilization.

Embryo transfer

Depending on your particular circumstances, your healthcare provider can help you determine if using fresh or frozen embryos is ideal for you. Both fresh and frozen embryo transfers follow the same protocol. The primary distinction is already apparent from the name. A fresh embryo transfer occurs three to seven days following the egg retrieval operation, when the embryo is put into your uterus. Since it hasn't been frozen, this embryo is "fresh." A frozen embryo transfer entails the thawing and implantation of frozen embryos (from an earlier IVF cycle or donor eggs) into your uterus. This method is increasingly popular due to practical reasons and the better chance of a live birth. Years after egg retrieval and fertilization can pass before frozen embryo transfers take place.

You will be given oral, injectable, vaginal, or trans-dermal hormones to get your uterus ready for receiving an embryo as part of the initial step in a frozen embryo transfer. Typically, this entails taking oral medication for 14 to 21 days, followed by injections for six days. You will often schedule two or three appointments during this time to assess your uterus' readiness using ultrasound and to measure your hormone levels using a blood test. You'll be scheduled for the embryo transfer process when your uterus is prepared.

When using fresh embryos, the procedure is similar, with the exception that the embryo transfer takes place three to five days after the embryo is removed. There is no need for anesthetic during the straightforward embryo transfer technique(If you've ever done a PAP test before this is almost similar to it). A tiny catheter is introduced into the uterus through the cervix using a speculum positioned within the vagina. A syringe with one or more embryos inside it is connected to the catheter's other end. Through the medium of the catheter the embryos are inserted into the uterus— the process usually takes less than ten minutes to complete.

Pregnancy

Pregnancy is the result you'd get from the embryo's integration with the uterine lining. About nine to fourteen days following embryo transfer, your doctor will perform a blood test to see if you're pregnant. If donor eggs are used, the same processes are performed. The egg donor in question will complete the ovarian stimulation and egg retrieval procedures. The embryo is transferred to the individual who will carry the pregnancy after fertilization (either with or without various fertility drugs). The success rate is dependent on a variety of variables, including the mother's age, the reason for her infertility, the condition of her embryos, her reproductive history, and her lifestyle choices. We discover that (IVF) applicants who are younger are more likely to become pregnant. A donor egg pregnancy is more likely in females over the age of 41. Women who have already given birth often have better (IVF) success rates than those who have never given birth(I guess experience is the best teacher after all).

So if you're worried about going through the (IVF) process I suggest you rest easy as the numbers are looking really up for those who have tried out the procedure. The only downsides to this is the cost and age factor. Even though one of the myths of the (IVF) people believe is that you can do the procedure at any age well that's not entirely true and we will talk about this in myth section below.

Popular Myths or Misconceptions IVF-Related

Well to be fair I did tell you earlier that the (IVF) wasn't magic right? But some people clearly believe that it is and it's this belief of theirs that has birthed some popular myths and misconceptions about the (IVF) procedure. Some of these myths sound completely nuts and unbelievable so we are only going to focus on the more sensible ones below;

Myth number one: The (IVF) is only for infertile couples

Although the (IVF) is often used to help a woman who otherwise can't conceive a child, you don't have to be infertile to benefit from (IVF). If you or your spouse have a genetic condition that could have an impact on the health and lifespan of your child, you may decide to use in vitro fertilization (IVF). And you have to admit this makes a lot more sense than believing that it is just for infertile women, seeing as we live in a world where currently genetic disorders from somewhere far up in the gene pool could creep up your baby unexpectedly the best bet you have to guard against this is the (IVF).

Myth number two: You can do the (IVF) at any age

No you cannot, time barely waits for anyone let alone for reproduction. If there's one thing that is trite is that as a woman ages, her reproductive system does too—with a particular focus on her egg quality.

Myth number three: (IVF) causes you to have multiple births

In order to maximize your chances of having a live birth, (IVF) labs used to frequently transfer a lot of viable embryos. However, in the decades that followed, technology improved. As a matter of fact, transferring multiple embryos may increase your chances of miscarriage or premature birth.

Myth number four: (IVF) is the only way to have a baby if you're infertile

You might not need (IVF) to have a healthy kid unless you or your partner have genetic difficulties or you two identify as same-sex partners. Only after you and your partner have undergone thorough fertility evaluations is recommend (IVF). Simpler methods, such surgery to correct structural issues or drugs to balance hormones, can be advantageous for you. Another option is artificial insemination, in which sperm from a donor or your spouse is inserted into your uterus without having a sexual encounter.

Myth number five: Fertility drugs cause cancer

It is trite that you must take drugs to trigger ovulation and the production of several eggs, but don't worry—they are harmless. More than 48.5 million couples around the world have used (IVF) to have a baby. But keep in mind that no research on health have found an elevated risk of cancer in the years following the treatment of these couples.

After diving deep into the intricacies of the (IVF) throughout this chapter if you still have doubts about it then look up what is possibly one of the best (IVF) success stories ever, about a sixty-seven year old female who is one of the oldest persons to go through the procedure in the African region by name Mrs. Ajibola Otunbusin. She and her spouse waited thirty-nine years to give birth and in the year 2018 she gave birth to a baby boy via the (IVF) procedure now tell me if that's not a scientific miracle.

CHAPTER FIVE
The Lifestyle Synopsis
(How Your Daily Habits Tend to Affect Your Fertility)

What you do, what you eat, and the activities that you engage in, play the most important role in determining how the general direction of your life flows in. I believe the old saying *"As you make your bed so shall you lie upon it"* comes into play here. This is an immutable fact of life and if your life habits are the general direction of your life then the area of your life that tethers on fertility isn't excluded as well.

Allow me to hypothetically bring before you two females and run a little bit of an experiment with them. Keep in mind that both are in their prime and both of them in the absence of any genetic disorder want to conceive. On one hand, we have the first female let's call her F1 and on the other hand, we have the second female called F2. The general lifestyle of F1 is centered on constant parties, smoking, and booze in Las Vegas every week not to mention the heavy intake of caffeine every morning to help with her hangovers.

F2 on the other hand understands the concept of *"taking a break"* She maintains a healthy diet abstains from alcohol or keeps it to a minimum at least and exercises whenever she can. These are the general lifestyles of these two females. Now, to the best of your reasoning who would among both of them have a higher chance of conceiving? Who among the both of them would likely produce higher quality eggs? Who has a lower risk of miscarriage or other pregnancy-related issues? If you have picked your winner then answer me this, why? What's the reason for your answer and why do you feel that the female you choose would have a better shot at conceiving than the other?

Sounds a bit nerdy right? I know, but I must give you my dear reader nothing less than the best. This chapter has made it its solemn duty to ensure that whatever lifestyle you have been living that affects your chances of conception is addressed and struck out. You will be educated on certain life habits that seem unimportant and casual but your fertility in a big way. You will be exposed to what you should cut out or stop doing to avoid fertility issues. And the best part of it all is that you will be taught how to improve your fertility levels both naturally and otherwise.

Shall we begin?

Lifestyle Vs Fertility

To be fertile means to reproduce. To be fertile means to wield the powers of creation in your body. When a woman conceives a child she touches the threshold of life—The child in her body is a sheer testament that life must continue on earth and the only beings in all of creation gifted this great power are the female folk nobody does it better than them and this is something that a woman mush take pride in for no matter how great and powerful a man can be he ultimately comes from a woman.

And so with this in mind infertility means existing in an unnatural state of being and your lifestyle could be a contributing factor to this unless you choose purposely not to give birth, but if you did you wouldn't be reading this book now would you? Female fertility as stated above is the ability of a female to bring forth a biological child and the best way to determine if you or your spouse have fertility issues is always to run a fertility test but before that, your first sign would be if you and your spouse have been having unprotected sex for six months and above and nothing happens. No results are seen, no miscarriages, no missed periods just nothing at this point you might not need a prophet to tell you that something's up.

In the absence of any known genetic disorders or hereditary issues, immutable factors like advanced age your best bet is to turn inwards and look at your life habits in-depth and there you might find the answer that you desire. Now that we stated this what those habits that's of ours that could affect fertility in females;

Chain smoking

While we do love to have a good smoke now and then putting a stop to your smoking lifestyle while trying to get pregnant will do you more good than you know. This is necessary because sometimes you might not even know that you're pregnant and I bet you did or didn't know that tobacco use is associated with lower fertility. If smoking in the United States or anywhere really has been flagged as one of the primal causes of health issues like lung cancer and chronic bronchitis what do you think it would do to your fertility and overall egg quality? But why wait Here's what smoking does to females it ages your ovaries and depletes your eggs prematurely I'm sure you get the big picture at this point so kindly put the cigarettes away. I am aware that most people can overcome their addiction to smoking, but if you are having trouble quitting, then you should seek your doctor for assistance.

Excessive caffeine consumption

I for one love the extra kick caffeine gives especially if I need to stay awake to finish a project or finish writing a book but I would not take caffeine excessively knowing fully well what it does to female fertility. Health experts advise though that you consider limiting your caffeine intake to one or two 6- to 8-ounce cups of coffee a day.

Overexercising

It is not bad to work out Trust me it is fun and those who here don't want to keep their bodies flexible and sexy but too much vigorous physical activity can inhibit ovulation and reduce the production of the hormone progesterone. Keep your weekly quantity of intense exercise to less than five hours if you are a healthy weight(obviously, we can't use the word 'fat' here but I'm sure you catch my drift) and intend to become pregnant soon.

Anovulation (a lack of ovulation) was shown to be more common in people who exercised for longer than 60 minutes per day, according to health reviews. What if I also told you that overdoing your exercise has a significant impact on your ovulation? Nevertheless, a compromise is made, and it is said that intense activity for 30 to 60 minutes each day decreases the chance of infertility brought on by anovulation.

Toxin inhalation

What if I told you that some of the most used items in our daily lives could harm your ability to conceive? Fertility can be negatively impacted by air fresheners, hand sanitizers, cleaning products, environmental contaminants, and poisons like pesticides, dry cleaning solvents, and lead. Before using these items, become a little bit of a geek and read the back labels for any potential chemicals utilized in said product that have the potential to influence your fertility or, worse still, induce miscarriages. The trick is in their level of toxicity.

Alcohol

Remember the illustration of F1 we gave earlier yeah? This life habit is based on her. While alcohol drinking is an age-long tradition almost as old as humanity itself, too much of everything is bad. Ovulation abnormalities are linked to an increased risk of heavy drinking. If you want to get pregnant, you might want to fully cut out alcohol. Since there is no known safe level of fetal alcohol consumption, abstinence is generally advised at conception and during pregnancy.

Special Exercise

After pointing out the above life habits I think it's best to leave it at this for now. The reason why these life habits were mentioned is that health reports show that they are the most common and somewhat difficult lifestyle habits to break out from and their impact on conception and pregnancy as a whole is drastic and thus they must be curtailed. If you have read up to this point I'd like you to go through these habits again and do two mental exercises.

- First, I want you to go through these habits again from a first-person point of view. Bearing in mind that the reason why I used the word "you" a lot when describing them is so you can personalize them, act on them, and know that if you're battling with any of these habits and you want to conceive then I'm talking to you here.

- Secondly, I want you to view these habits from a third-person point of view. Think of yourself as a wise and experienced master advising a student. Once you have done this ask yourself what habits are I struggling with so badly. Can I let them go? Do I want to be fertile and conceive along the way? Or do I just don't care about whatever health and fertility impacts that my lifestyle has on me?

Take two deep breathes and take a space of about five minutes to ponder on this, You don't have to be in a quiet space or special position (although they would help a lot) you just have to make sure that your mind is actively thinking about what you want and what is best for you.

Lifestyle Vs Fertility (Premium Fertility Booster)

The entirety of this chapter is based on two things, (in between clearing any doubts that come up as it regards fertility), It consists of what you should stop doing that affects your fertility and what you should do that would help boost your fertility it is as simple as that. It is trite that there's always light at the end of the proverbial tunnel for those who believe, Having pointed out the life habits that negatively impact fertility in females let's bring out the best and talk about those lifestyle habits that if aren't already doing that you should do more to boost your fertility and aid in conception as a female.

Let's begin, shall we?

Just sleep

Every element of our life is impacted by sleep. Lack of sleep can have an impact on how well we perform at work and in school, it can influence our judgment and mood, and it can even result in long-term health issues. Insufficient sleep can also have an impact on fertility. Although the exact cause of this is unknown, health professionals speculate that hypothalamic pituitary adrenal (HPA) activation and circadian dysrhythmia may obstruct reproduction. Additionally, a small review of research discovered that women who worked fixed night shifts saw a slight rise in miscarriage rates. All genders may develop excess weight as a result of poor sleep. Ovulation issues might result from severe extra weight. Additionally, obesity and excess weight might affect the health of sperm.

If you're seriously considering conception and you want a way to get the best out of your sleep game then you might want to consider trying out the simple and easy-to-follow list below;

- Stick to a set sleep and wake schedule.
- Follow a nightly bedtime routine.
- Get adequate daylight exposure and physical activity.
- TVs, phones, and laptops should not be used in the bedroom.
- Keep caffeine, alcohol, and heavy meals away from bedtime.
- Create a peaceful resting environment in your bedroom.

Exercise regularly

To be clear I don't mean strenuous exercises like lifting above your weight, boxing classes, and mountain climbing(you're not in the WWE, even if you're I don't think Brie and Nikki Bella did all of that stuff while they were trying to conceive). Your immune system, heart, and lungs will all benefit from exercise. Regular exercise might be crucial for those who are obese or overweight. Regardless of a person's weight, health research has shown that physical activity marginally increases the likelihood of getting pregnant in one menstrual cycle. Remember that if you must exercise as an adult, you should aim for at least 150 to 300 minutes a week of moderate-intensity exercise and two days of muscle-strengthening exercises, per the 2018 Physical Activity Guidelines for Americans.

Make a habit of testing yourself regularly

By testing here I mean health tests. It's not a good idea to always walk around like you're the female version of Clark Kent whose health is powered by the sun. As humans, we have health issues now and then however slight is part of our biological composition so unless you have cells made of steel I advise that you schedule a visit to your health provider now and then to check up to ensure that all systems are good to go. This is especially important when you're trying to conceive You might want to run fertility tests, tests on STIs and STDs, and even tests that would help ascertain any fertility affecting-genetic disorder, this helps to know your medical standing and acts as a confidence booster to your chances of conception.

Avoid alcohol and smoking

I feel as though we have pointed out all we need to know about the adverse impacts alcohol and smoking have on fertility when we talked about the negative life habits earlier but I just couldn't help but stress on this one more time. Stating it plainly that alcohol and smoking are bad for the fertility business and they have even worse effects on the egg quality of the female and based on this it's a no-brainer that avoiding them entirely or at least during the period that you are trying to conceive is going to boost your chances.

Eating a healthy diet

One must never underestimate the power of a healthy meal. When trying to increase fertility, conceive, or even just stay healthy during pregnancy, nutrition can be very effective. According to health studies, diets high in whole grains, fruits, vegetables, fish, and unsaturated fats are linked to increased fertility in all genders, not just women. The U.S. Department of Agriculture recommends consuming 85% of daily calories from nutrient-dense foods and 15% of calories from added sugars and saturated fats.

Don't worry no one is asking you to stick to a monk-like meal plan although you can do it if that's what you want though(just kidding). It's best you keep one thing in mind, eat but don't eat excessively Trust me you do not want to become obese from eating junk meals and you do not want to find out what effects excessive obesity has on fertility. Keep your eyes on awesome meals like the amazing pear and cheese breakfast sandwich, stuffed acorn squash, or even a crab salad sandwich if you're into sea foods — the nutritional properties of these simple meals and a lot more like them are off the charts and how do I know this, well in addition to being heavily health and nutrition oriented I have one more secret(I'm a huge foodie).

CHAPTER SIX
The Power in Nutrition
(A Dietary Guide You'd Want to Follow For Enhanced Egg Quality)

If you have never been a fan of the old saying about *"you being what you eat"* then kindly permit me to change your mind on that, because if you don't believe this then you're seriously underestimating the power of nutrition. Let's say two men are walking down the street on a very hot summer afternoon and one of them just had the worst burger under the heavens he's grumpy about his violated taste buds and just wants to go home. The other just had some delicious iced tea, is in a fairly good mood, and might even be signing as well. And then came along you who mistakenly bumps into both of them. Now, in this situation who do you think is more likely to give you an earful among the two men(I let you figure this one out genius).

Food is good and good food is powerful. It is one of the places where my nutrition company draws its awesome catchphrase (you'll find out about that more in the future). Did you know that food can affect not just your physical aspects but also your mental aspects Food can make you grateful, satisfied, and happy but a meal that's so bad that it reminds you of a funeral will leave both you, your mind, and your palate feeling bereaved.

If nutrition has such power and affects us all in various aspects then it no doubt has an impact on fertility with particular reference to enhancing the egg quality of females to promote higher conception chances. Have you ever heard of something called Tiger Nuts before? (And no I don't mean the actual nuts of a tiger, lord no!) It's a tiny fruit that grows in the African region that can be chewed directly or processed into milk and when the milk is consumed by the male spouse his seed becomes so potent that there are reports of birthing twins at a single go.

Pretty interesting stuff right? But that would be useful if we were talking about the fertility of the males but nope, I humbly dedicate this chapter on dietary nutrition to the females who need a boost in the quality of their eggs. Two things come into play here what you should eat to enhance your egg quality and what you should not eat or stop eating entirely so it doesn't cause negative effects on the quality of your eggs. To put this simply we are going to be talking about food lots of it. Food as it concerns the meals that you eat, the fruits that you take, and the supplements that you consume. Everything is vital and everything has to be considered on the path to improving egg quality no stone should be left unturned so let's begin.

Egg Quality Nutrition;Harmful Dietary Patterns

Before you begin your egg nutrition journey you must be sure of two things; first, be sure about the quality of your eggs, and second you need to understand what a bad quality egg is and its signs and symptoms. The reason for this is simple, it is to ensure that you don't panic unnecessarily if you can't conceive quickly because not everyone is built the same and these things take a while sometimes. And, so that you don't go spending hundreds of dollars on medical procedures when there's nothing wrong with you. So with that in mind let's answer the question, What is a bad egg quality? Low egg quality is frequently referred to as "diminished ovarian reserve," which causes female infertility. Age is the main factor contributing to low egg quality, but there are other causes as well, such as pelvic radiation, ovarian surgery, any reproductive ailment, genetic abnormalities, chemotherapy, excessive nicotine and alcohol usage, and other unidentified variables.

Aging raises the risk of ovulation with eggs of inferior quality and increases the likelihood of miscarriage. The biggest barrier to fertilization is poor egg quality, which also causes issues during implantation and development. Although it's generally accepted that older women have eggs of lower quality, it has occasionally been seen that younger women can experience infertility at a young age and have eggs of lower quality as well. As a result, it's critical to pay attention to your body's changes and recognize the signs that your eggs' quality is declining.

Speaking of symptoms these are some of the signs and symptoms that you'd want to keep an eye out for if you find yourself subject to any of them;

- Complexity in getting pregnant.
- Late or no periods at all.
- Shorter menstrual cycle than usual.
- Miscarriage.
- Heavy menstrual flow.

Now it doesn't necessarily mean that once a woman has some of these symptoms she automatically has bad egg quality, Recall what I said earlier not everyone is built the same and thus what might be a symptom to one lady might not be a symptom to you. But your best bet is if you see any of these go run a medical test with a trusted health provider just to be sure before you proceed to take the next line of action.

What about the meals, fruits, or supplements? What about those things that you consume that negatively affect your egg quality? You'll find the answer to this question in the list below;

Sugar-sweetened beverages

One health study looked at the reproductive impacts of drinking sugar-sweetened beverages for periods of up to 12 menstrual cycles among 3,828 females aged 21 to 45 and 1,045 of their male partners who were planning pregnancies. Regular usage of sugar-sweetened beverages, which is defined as consuming at least 7 drinks per week, has been linked to decreased fertility in both males and females, according to health researchers.

Compared to diet sodas and fruit juice, which revealed no discernible link to fertility, sugar-sweetened sodas and energy drinks had the worst impact. Another health study discovered that women's overall numbers of mature and fertilized eggs and high-quality embryos were lower when they drank more sugary beverages. This appeared to have a stronger negative effect on fertility than caffeinated beverages without added sugar and was irrespective of the amount of caffeine present. But despite this, drinking soda is linked to lower fertility. Try seltzer water or normal water that has been organically flavored with lemon slices or berries as an alternative to sugary drinks.

Certain dairy products

Dairy fat intake seems to have sex-specific impacts on fertility. According to certain health studies, whole milk may boost female fertility whereas low-fat dairy products may be optimal for promoting male fertility. According to a 2007 health study, low-fat dairy products were linked to an increased risk of infertility, but high-fat dairy products were linked to a lower chance of ovulation-related infertility. When compared to women who consumed full-fat dairy products less frequently, at about once a week, they had a 25% lower risk of fertility problems related to ovulatory disorders. In addition, compared to women who consumed low-fat dairy only once a week, those who consumed more than two servings per day were 85% more likely to have infertility as a result of a lack of ovulation. Instead of consuming dairy products, you may choose a choice of plant-based milk, cheese, and dairy products with varied fat contents.

Baked goods

A lot of trans and saturated fats can be found in baked pastries, donuts, and cakes, especially if they have been fried or contain margarine. Consuming these lipids is linked to less successful female conception. You might be surprised to learn that when manufacturers partially hydrogenate vegetable oils to make them solid at room temperature, trans fats are created. Despite being formally outlawed from the food supply as of January 20, 2021, goods with less than 0.5 grams of trans fat per serving can still be marked as such.

Fertility issues have been associated with diets that are high in trans fats and low in unsaturated fats. This is especially true for diets where trans fats account for more than 1% of total calories. Additionally, trans fat consumption is linked to a 73% increased chance of ovulatory problems, which can result in infertility, according to a health study. In conclusion, diets that prioritize monounsaturated fats over trans fats are linked to better reproductive results.

Vitamin A

We have vitamin A in the category of supplements, and this is crucial for the health of your immune system, reproductive system, eyes, and other major organs. However, health professionals have warned that it can have disastrous effects if taken in excessive doses, such as before something as straightforward as outpatient elective surgery. Vitamin A, especially its derivatives, should be avoided when trying to conceive when it comes to fertility specifically. The National Institutes of Health state that ingesting too much vitamin A during the first trimester of pregnancy (more than the advised 770 mcg RAE) has been linked to congenital birth problems like deformities of the heart, lungs, eyes, and skull.

Mega nutrients

If you're trying to conceive in one place don't want to find yourself in a place where you lack the necessary nutrients to build your egg quality up. However, doing this is certainly not your best bet. Mega nutrients that seemingly appear to be harmless, when consumed by a woman trying to conceive could prove disastrous since they contain very high levels of certain nutrients that are quite harmful to female fertility. If you're lost in thoughts about this don't be, do one simple thing and that's sticking to a healthier meal and you're good to go.

But something's missing here. What about fruits that you should avoid? Certain fruits should not be taken if you're trying to conceive and they shouldn't even be taken while you're pregnant as well and among the possibly hundreds of fruits out there three of them made it to the top of that list.

Here they are;

Pineapple

Although pineapples are typically healthy to eat, I wouldn't advise pregnant women to consume them if they're seeking to improve the quality of their eggs. They may trigger premature contractions because they include enzymes that change the smoothness of the cervix. This might result in a miscarriage. It is also known to cause diarrhea, which can be very uncomfortable during pregnancy. Consider them to be the one fruit you enjoy eating every day of the week 'except' when you are trying to conceive or pregnant.

Papaya

It shouldn't come as a surprise that papaya ranks first on this list. However, the situation with papayas is a little unique. Papayas that are raw or semi-ripe contain latex, which might harm your unborn child and trigger early labor. On the other hand, ripe papaya is rich in vitamins and iron. While consuming unripe papaya while trying to improve the quality of your eggs or while pregnant is not advised, doing so in moderation won't hurt you.

Grapes

Grapes are delicious no doubt and sometimes when I eat them it makes me feel like Roman royalty but they are not recommended for consumption when trying to improve egg quality and during the third trimester of pregnancy. They are known to produce heat in the body, which harms both the mother and the child. To put this graphically it is almost like cooking your eggs or fetus while inside your body so to avoid complications, avoid eating too many grapes before and during pregnancy.

Egg Quality Nutrition; Dietary Patterns that Boost Fertility

There's hardly anyone on the planet who doesn't want to improve in one way or the other in any area or aspects of their lives, the same applies to women who want to be more fertile to increase their chances of conception. We have talked about the majority of the things that you should steer clear from consuming if you don't want any issues when it comes to conceiving, now it's time for the fun part which is, what you should eat to boost your egg fertility.

You should start simple don't overdo it or rush but start by adding a bit by bit daily some of the meals, fruits, and supplements to be mentioned below just so long as you don't have any medical allergies that prevent you from eating them. Let's begin;

Antioxidants

The antioxidants are first on this list since they are essential for shielding an egg's developing shell from harm. In a follicle filled with follicular fluid, the egg grows. Antioxidants ought to be abundant in this liquid. While vitamin C and vitamin E have more immediate antioxidant effects, minerals like zinc and selenium are components of antioxidant molecules. If you consume little fruits, vegetables, nuts, and seeds in your diet, you may be deficient in antioxidants. If you are worried about the quality of your eggs, you should concentrate on these highly important food groups.

Zinc

One of the body's most prevalent antioxidant molecules is zinc. Zinc deficiency is a widespread condition that frequently manifests. Meat, chickpeas, almonds, and seeds all contain zinc. However, absorption might be challenging, putting people who have weak digestion in jeopardy. Mal-absorption is a danger for people using long-term proton pump inhibitors (PPI), which are frequently recommended stomach acid inhibitors. Additionally, persons who consume a lot of plants may also be in danger unless measures are taken to improve dietary absorption, such as soaking, sprouting, and fermenting.

Selenium

One significant family of antioxidant proteins includes selenium. Selenium is abundant in Brazil nuts, yet it is simple to consume too much of it. Consume Brazil nuts occasionally, but not too frequently, as just one nut might supply more than the daily required amount. The amount of selenium in the soil near your home or the source of your animal products can affect whether you have a selenium shortage. Selenium is also present in beef, chicken, fish, shellfish, and eggs.

Vitamin C and E

These antioxidants are crucial, especially for women over 35. Together, they promote fertility. Fresh fruits and vegetables contain vitamin C, thus health professionals advise consuming 2 pieces of fruit and 5 meals of vegetables each day. Almonds, avocados, sunflower seeds, salmon, sweet potatoes, olives, and olive oil all contain vitamin E. If you take supplements, you may only be high in one type of vitamin E as a result.

Vitamin B6 and vitamin B12

Together, these two vitamins manage a healthy hormone balance and start ovulation on schedule, which can increase your chances of getting pregnant. The proper dosage of B6 aids in the promotion of balanced levels of progesterone and estrogen, which are essential for the cell signaling that occurs during ovulation and egg development. The production of healthy blood and cell division both require vitamin B12. Supplementing these critical vitamins at amounts supported by research also improves (IVF) results.

Folate

This protects against protects against chromosomal abnormalities. Chromosome abnormalities in the egg that develop during maturation are a common cause of infertility, miscarriage, and unsuccessful IVF rounds. Supplementing with high-quality, methylated folate has been shown to substantially lower the risk of chromosomal abnormalities. Additionally, having enough folate can increase your chances of getting pregnant, allowing you to have a child sooner.

That's about enough with the supplements and nutrients part now let's go to the area of meals and fruits.

Sunflower seeds

My favorite kind of seeds are sunflower seeds. Sunflower seed kernels that have been roasted and left unsalted are high in vitamin E, a necessary component that has been found to increase sperm count and motility in certain men. Selenium and folate, which are critical for both male and female reproduction, are also abundant in sunflower seeds. In addition to being a strong supply of omega-6 fatty acids, sunflower seeds also contain tiny levels of omega-3 fatty acids, which are incredibly significant. Sprinkle them on your favorite salads or dishes, then relax and indulge.

Well-aged cheese

Cheese that has matured or been aged well is rich in polyamines, which are proteins that may be found in both plant and animal products. They also exist in humans naturally. According to medical studies, polyamines may be crucial to the reproductive system. The polyamine putrescine, which may be important for sperm health, is particularly abundant in mature cheese. Additionally, putrescine may enhance egg health, particularly in women over 35. Although it is nutrient-rich and helps to improve egg quality, occasionally a patient has complained of a cheese allergy, so keep in mind what I said earlier: if you fall into any of these categories, avoid your allergies and explore other ways to do so since there are so many available.

Liver

One of the foods on the Planet with the highest nutrients per serving is liver, especially cow's liver. There are many fat-soluble vitamins in it, including vitamin A, which is hard to find in other parts of the diet. In addition to being the best natural source of vitamin A, the liver is also a rich supply of vitamin B12, necessary for the correct synthesis of DNA and red blood cells, and highly absorbable iron, which helps avoid miscarriage and maternal anemia. Additionally, choline, omega-3 fatty acids, and folate are abundant in the liver.

Egg Yolks

The yolk of an egg contains the majority of the egg's iron, calcium, zinc, vitamin B6, folate, and vitamin B12 content. They also include all of the vitamin A found in eggs. Egg yolks from chickens fed on pasture are also rich in fat-soluble vitamins A, D, E, and K2 as well as omega-3 fatty acids EPA and DHA, which support fertility. Eggs are a cheap source of lean protein, which is beneficial for both men's and women's fertility. This makes them a healthy food choice. Choline, which is also found in eggs, may lower the incidence of various birth abnormalities. Not all research, nevertheless, has discovered this advantage.

Berries

Berries like raspberries, blueberries, and strawberries all have anti-inflammatory phytonutrients and natural antioxidants, two elements that significantly enhance the quality of eggs.

Avocados

And last on this list is the legendary avocados. I feel like the importance of avocados has been grossly underestimated While they may not have overly attractive exteriors like exotic fruits like apples and grapes there is hardly a nutritional recommendation that you'd receive out there that doesn't contain avocados. They are rich in monounsaturated fatty acids, vitamin A, and folate, which promote reproductive health, and not very many fruits can top that.

If we decided to list every single supplement, every single fruit, and every single meal that is required to boost female egg quality we would fill this entire book up and still be looking for extra pages to add still. The above is not an exclusive list but we certainly made sure that we presented before you the most important ones.

With that being said, cheers to your healthier nutritional life.

CHAPTER SEVEN
Medical Breakthroughs
(Contemporary Innovations and Discoveries in Fertility Treatment)

Did you know that in almost every area of our lives, there are always constant variables? Let me explain why, If you go online today you'll find that are always arguments about politics right? There are also heated discussions about which religion is best, then there is the area of morality and ethics people constantly bicker about what is right and what is wrong to no end. But one of the most constant variables is technology and science has been ignored for decades until recently. Borrowing the words of Carl Sagan here *"We live in a society exquisitely dependent on science and technology, in which hardly anyone knows anything about science and technology."* With this in mind, it can be said that in this current time and age, there is hardly an area of life in which science and technology don't play a vital role in fertility.

It was a scientific breakthrough in the medical field that gave us the cesarean operation or c-section for short to help mothers who couldn't conceive naturally. It gave us incubation to cater for premature babies or babies born under special circumstances and today scientific and technological breakthroughs have given us the in-vitro fertilization (IVF) which is nothing short of a scientific miracle.

We can't begin to count how many couples have had their hearts broken in the past due to infertility or barrenness. To every good couple out there, a child or children are a source of joy and a chance for their legacy on earth to continue but barrenness and infertility made that wish a pipe dream for so many years. But today and in the future, technological advancements and scientific breakthroughs in the medical field have made that desire a reality burning to ashes the verdict of barrenness and telling you that yes, you can conceive so long as you're in the right place. That hopeless situation of childlessness is now a hopeful situation filled with children.

So now we ask the question, what are these so-called fertility advancements in the medical field? How effective are they? Do they work for everyone? Are there any defects or side effects? And what does the future hold for technologically-inspired fertility? We will spend a greater part of this chapter tackling these questions and more and at the end, you're sure to be more inspired than troubled if you have any issues fertility-related.

Fertility Vs. Science and Technology; How Far We Have Come

If there is an area that mankind has relentlessly poured in their efforts it's the medical field people want to live longer dealing with mortality issues, mothers want to conceive healthier babies who live longer and are free of genetic disorders, and expectant mothers want to be more fertile and science and cutting edge technology has made this possible in so many ways. Since the groundbreaking development of in-vitro fertilization (IVF) in the 1970s, infertility has surprisingly seen little innovation, despite being a highly common sickness (yep, anything that makes you feel uneasy is a disease). Due to the extremely difficult-to-modulate biological pathways and the regulatory, legal, and ethical constraints on research, development, and commercialization, innovation in this field is frequently tough. However, several fertility breakthrough innovations are currently being developed that have the potential to drastically alter both the lives of many couples and society as a whole.

Infertility affects more women of reproductive age than cancer, diabetes, or high blood pressure combined. Over 100 million people worldwide struggle with infertility, with one in eight couples reportedly having trouble getting pregnant. It is common knowledge that age and infertility go hand in hand. While the U.S. infertility rate for women 30-34 years old was 14% in 2018, it was already more than double for women 35-39 years old (39%) and almost 50% for women 40-44 years old (48%) in 2018. Therefore, population dynamics and epidemiological changes are important causes of infertility. The average age at childbirth has significantly increased, especially in the West, as families are choosing to have children later in life. From 1997 to 2017, the percentage of American women giving birth between the ages of 45 and 49 increased by an astonishing 125%, that between the ages of 40 and 44 by 63%, and that between the ages of 35 and 39 by 47%.

Additionally, biological factors including the increased incidence of obesity, which increases ovulation infertility and poor sperm count, have an impact on infertility rates. Having stated this I find that two huge questions get asked a lot and they are Can infertility be cured? And how common is infertility? For now, there isn't any written-in-stone answer or a concrete response to that question but one thing I can tell you is that in addition to you doing your part and cutting off any live habits that affect your egg quality, your fertility clinic will first of all address any underlying issues you have this is where the fertility test comes in to determine the state of your reproductive system. Then if you're the type who is constantly exposed to harmful environmental toxins the fertility facility would recommend ways to avoid them before the actual fertilization treatments would begin.

This is logical because in this situation if you're undergoing fertility treatments and you're still engaging in activities that hinder fertility then you're going to get slower results. To answer the next question you get a resounding yes I can give you more than one answer as to why infertility is quite common. Infertility is quite common it is almost as common as how men in their youth experience the receding of their hairlines which eventually leads to frontal baldness if not taken care of properly. But the thing is that most females are ignorant of this or choose not to pay attention to it until they find themselves running from pillar to post seeking ways to boost their fertility or to conceive.

The second reason that infertility is common is that most females are of the old beliefs and would rather have children naturally against all odds than undergo assisted reproduction. They view this from a moral standpoint and question the ethics of having a child through (IVF) or even through surrogacy and a key factor here is that some of them might be from families that have strong beliefs that kick against modern scientific and technological techniques that assists in conception.

Then there is the issue of laws it is widely known thing that the laws of all the countries of the world are not the same; for instance, the United States and Canada may agree on some universal laws but ultimately they don't agree on the same set of laws don't be surprised if you come across a country where certain medical procedure are banned there.

And most importantly in addition to not having adequate awareness about the assisted reproductive technology out there, money comes into consideration and this is something I made clear in previous chapters. For a procedure as complex as assisted reproduction being cheap isn't an option. Let's take (IVF) as an example; it frequently has hefty expenses and is not covered by health insurance in many nations. While the national median income is only about $61,000, the average cost of a (IVF) cycle in the U.S. is about $23,000. Couples typically need 2.3–2.7 cycles, which results in a total average cost of $53,000–65,000. Are these fertility treatments effective? Yes no doubt there are, If a 67-year-old female could give birth through (IVF) then that speaks volumes of its effectiveness but ultimately it deepens on two things your budget and your age. Having pointed this out it is only fair that we survey the fertility innovations that modern science and technology have brought our way with the exclusion of the (IVF) they include;

Treatment with gonadotropins

These medications support women who ovulate irregularly or before the egg is fully developed. When a woman ovulates, the pituitary gland modifies the timing to ensure a mature ovum.

During in vitro fertilization, certain women might get letrozole and gonadotropin therapy.

Infertility treatments with clomid

By causing ovulation in females who do not produce an egg, this medicine also interacts with the pituitary gland to work. Increased live birth rates are the outcome of enhanced ovarian response to follicle-stimulating hormone (FSH) following treatment with Clomid.

Infertility treatments with letrozole

Letrozole is used to treat post-menopausal women with breast cancer. It suppresses the production of estrogen, which has an impact on the pituitary and hypothalamus' ability to regulate ovulation (National Institutes of Health). Women with PCOS may benefit greatly from letrozole's potential for conception assistance.

Of all the recent advancements and breakthroughs in the field of fertility, these are by far the most successful ones besides (IVF) Each of these innovations is designed to combat and remedy a specific area of infertility-related issues and that's not even half of it the future of the medical field and what is to come will be sure to leave your jaw-dropping.

Fertility vs the Future; How Far Will We Go?

With the speed of technological innovations these days the future is sure to hit you faster than you can say great Scott! One of the only factors that hinder these technological advancements in fertility is laws. It is no news that laws are based on morality, ethics, political and social considerations as regards the general populace living in that geographical area. Before a law is passed regarding areas as complex as health and life in general it is always a very complicated process.

In the U.S. today there is still much controversial dust as it regards abortion laws and the same applies to fertility laws but the thing is, time waits for no one and while arguments and debates are being held as to what laws would be good for whom and what fertility treatments they should consider some other countries don't care much for these technicalities and are moving at a rather fast pace — a good example of this would be the UK who are moving so fast in the medical field that many other countries can only eat their dust.

Here's a sneak peek at what the future of fertility treatments holds;

Lab-grown eggs and sperm

The ability to produce eggs and sperm in a lab setting is significantly improving thanks to scientific advancements. The end goal is to take adult skin cells, turn them into "induced pluripotent stem cells" that can differentiate into different cell types, and then use a chemical cocktail to guide these cells down the developmental pathway to become either eggs or sperm cells.

Although this may seem biologically impossible, researchers have already succeeded in creating healthy offspring in mice. It would be revolutionary if a sperm cell could be created from a female skin cell and vice versa. It is difficult to translate this work into human cells. There are still significant scientific obstacles to clear, and proving safety would take time. However, there is rising optimism that this may ultimately be viable, and businesses are actively working to introduce the most recent innovations to reproductive clinics.

Human genome editing

Yes, sir, you heard me correctly; if this is a tremendous success, you can bid genetic and inherited abnormalities farewell in the future. Genome editing is a technique for changing a cell's or an organism's DNA in a precise way. Genetic illnesses are currently treated in medicine via gene therapy, which involves adding new genes or disabling defective genes in particular cells. The genetic alterations would take place in every cell of the body and be passed on to succeeding generations if the DNA of an embryo were altered. The method might make it possible to prevent the spread of heritable disorders. However, we are still a few years away from this breakthrough because of the precise needs of the operation, not to mention the pre-implantation of embryos and getting the genome editing perfect to avoid any unintended outcomes. Nevertheless, this is undoubtedly something to look forward to.

Three-person baby (IVF)

The most significant change to UK fertility regulations occurred in 2015 as a result of a vote to permit a procedure known as mitochondrial transfer, which is intended to cure some fatal genetic illnesses. The procedure entails replacing the egg's mitochondrial DNA, which makes up a very small portion of the total DNA and is located outside the egg's nucleus, with donor DNA from a healthy person. Only two specific methods are now allowed, but many individuals want the rule to be more open-ended so that additional methods with the same goal might be licensed. Future expansion of the technique's uses is conceivable, and this could lead to a wide range of fertility-related outcomes.

Synthetic embryos

Pause for a minute here, Have you seen the old movie Man of Steel which starred Henry Cavill? There was a scene there where the reproductive process of the people of Krypton was explained and how they were designed with synthetic embryos — with each embryo being fine-tuned to a specific purpose like how the main villain General Zod was designed to be a soldier his whole life, with the potential that lies in synthetic embryos this would no longer exist only in the movies but would soon become reality. Currently, the UK has guidelines governing the use of embryos in research that limit how far along in development they can be cultured in the lab to 14 days. According to health reports, scientific teams are working to develop these embryo-like entities from mouse cells, complete with a beating heart and primitive brain. The artificial embryos are virtually identical to "real" embryos in appearance, but they cannot be created with an egg or sperm. To gain a deeper understanding of human development, including why many pregnancies end prematurely, these same scientists are attempting to replicate the work in human cells. If this technological improvement makes a significant breakthrough, there will be fewer miscarriage problems and more births in the future.

Technology is constantly on the move never resting and always advancing in the fight against infertility in more ways than one and I bet you that even at the time of writing this book there are still more innovations being made and more breakthroughs coming through it is only a matter of time before the future arrives—but on till then the best thing to do is make use of available advancements and scientific opportunities fertility-related to better both your life and the life of your spouse.

CHAPTER EIGHT
Craving Out Your Story
(Personal Paths Through Fertility)

I'd like you to think of this last chapter as not a chapter but a conversation between us both based on realities not just mere facts. Allow me to tell you a little tale, years ago A young mother(as she was then) had her first child through a C-section a healthy baby boy which was good and then she had her second baby boy through another C-section since she had a narrow pelvis issue but due to genetic anomalies which caused some health complications the baby passed away shortly and that was it for her— she couldn't conceive again for the rest of her life.

Not a single day goes by that the memory of that loss doesn't replay in her head as she ponders what could have been or how old he would have been— all those thoughts fill her mind even after so long has passed. But the truth is, life must go on however painful it might be(at this point I'm pretty sure that whoever is reading this can already tell who the young mother in the quote is). Sometimes we are dealt cards that we don't want to play and sometimes we don't always get what we want so badly but the bottom line is, so long as there are other options then you should go for those other options so you don't become tethered to an obsession that starts fine but later becomes unhealthy.

In the neighborhood I grew up in, one of my favorites Aunts at the time and friend of the family let's call her Aunt.N who was and is very pretty got married early on and a few years later I left that neighborhood with my family for a fresh start but almost ten years after that when we heard from Aunt.N she still hadn't conceived and in the end she resulted to adoption when all else had proved uneventful and today she's a happy mother. If there's one thing that inspired me about her at the time I'd have to say it was her mindset— she never let her situation weigh her down or make her grumpy.

She was always cheerful and had a smile on, despite feeling that emptiness of not having a child and to make matters worse scientific and technological innovations weren't as advanced then as there are now and the level of awareness on (IVF) was as poor as a church rat — she didn't have the opportunity many of you reading this have right now to be blessed with an era that is filled with so many options and opportunities that are offered by new innovations but she had hope.

My reason for telling you this is to advise you to always have hope despite the situations and trials that you might find yourself going through fertility-wise, even if it seems like there is no light at the end of the tunnel your resilience will speak for you. I believe it was Mickey Rooney that said *"You will always pass failure on your way to success."* while this is true the main heroine of the story is you and the level of resilience that you show on your way determines your success.

Success is achievable even after all the initial set back, a prime example of this is the success story of the 38 year old female called patient X and her 40 year old spouse who were able to still conceive after seven years of marriage (as reported by the Nova (IVF) fertility center). Her case wasn't an easy one it took multiple (IVF) cycles and multiple procedures were employed to get the job done but in the end the job was done and today she's a proud mom.

In addition to a positive mindset on these matters I advise that you take care of yourself both physically and mentally as well — this is part of the reason why I included the chapter on lifestyle habits because I want you to be in the best shape of your life before undergoing any medical procedures if you so desire. Remember a healthy body and a healthy mind make up a healthy person so don't go beating yourself up and sinking into depression if things don't go the way you want at the first instance when there is always room for seconds.

It is my desire that you keep an eye on your mental health throughout your fertility journey. it is also my desire that you maintain a positive mindset and very vividly define what your own success is. Sometimes success isn't defined by a successful pregnancy but I have heard stories of people who find their successes in finding closure, moving on or choosing another path to parenthood like surrogacy or adoption. One way or the other it is my desire for you that your days be filled with happiness and whatever fertility issues you might have become a thing of the past.

Cheer to your fruitful life!

Kathie.

COURSE UQ FOR VISIONARY LEADERS

Lesson 1 - Balancing Potentials

KATIA DORIA FONSECA VASCONCELOS